# BANANA: COLORFUL, BRIGHT AND HEALTHY

*Amazing health benefits of Banana*

**By**

Mercy Obidake

Table of contents

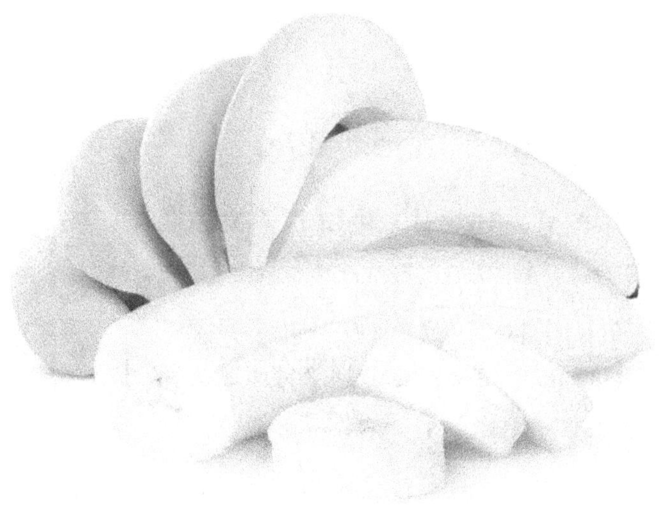

## Introduction

Bananas are tasty and have a lovely appearance. Aside from these, they also have several health benefits. They contain several nutrients which enhances our body's performance. This book covers the nutrients and various health benefits of banana. Also, a special tutorial on how to prepare banana smoothie which is also very nutritious is contained in this book.

# Chapter One

## The banana plant

The banana is botanically a berry produced by different kinds of large herbaceous flowering plants in the genus Musa. It is an edible fruit. In some countries, banana is used for cooking and often referred to as plantains.

Banana is variable in color, size and firmness, but is usually curved and elongated, with a soft flesh, which may be yellow, green, purple, red, or brown when ripe.

Almost all modern bananas come from two wild species known as Musa acuminata and Musa balbisiana.

The largest herbaceous flowering plant is the banana. Banana plants are usually tall and fairly sturdy, often mistaken for trees, however, what looks a trunk is just a pseudostem or "false stem". Bananas thrive in a wide variety of soils, 60 cm deep, have a great drainage and are not compacted.

# Chapter two

## Nutrients in Banana

There are several health benefits of banana and this is traceable to the nutrients the fruit contains. The following are several nutrients found in a banana.

## Vitamins

Choline 9.8 mg
Niacin 0.665 mg 3 %
Folate 20.00 mcg
Betaine 0.1 mg
Pantothenic acid 0.334 mg 3 %
Thiamin 0.031 mg 2 %
Riboflavin 0.073 mg 4 %
Vitamin A, RAE 3.00 mcg
Vitamin A 64.00 IU 1 %
Carotene, beta 26.00 mcg
Lutein + zeaxanthin 22.00 mcg
Carotene, alpha 25.00 mcg

Vitamin B6 0.367 mg 18 %

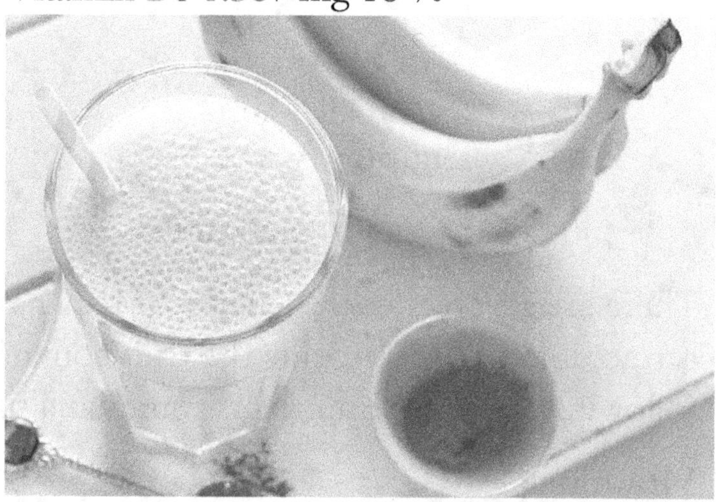

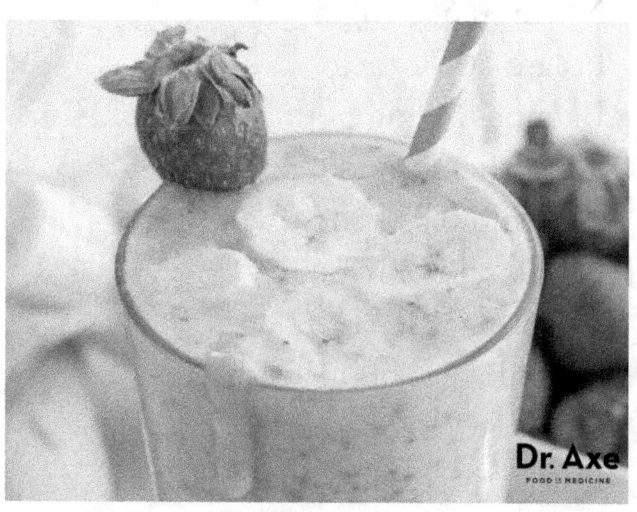

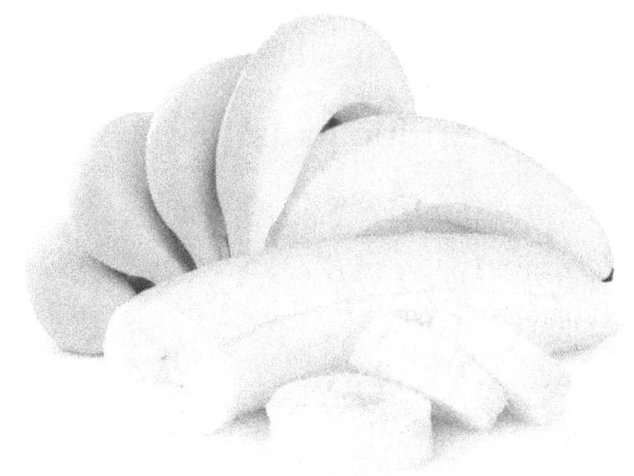

Vitamin E 0.10 mg 0 %
Vitamin C 8.7 mg 14 %
Tocopherol, alpha 0.10 mg
Tocopherol, gamma 0.02 mg
Tocopherol, delta 0.01 mg
Tocotrienol, alpha 0.06 mg
Vitamin K 0.5 mcg 1 %

## Minerals

Copper, Cu 0.078 mg 4 %
Calcium, Ca 5.00 mg 0 %
Iron, Fe 0.26 mg 1 %
Fluoride, F 2.2 mcg
Manganese, Mn 0.270 mg 14 %
Phosphorus, P 22.00 mg 2 %
Magnesium, Mg 27.00 mg 7 %
Selenium, Se 1.0 mcg 1 %
Sodium, Na 1.00 mg 0 %

Potassium, K 358.00 mg 8 %
Zinc, Zn 0.15 mg 1 %

## Proteins and Aminoacids

Alanine 0.040 g
Protein 1.09 g 2 %
Aspartic acid 0.124 g
Arginine 0.049 g
Glutamic acid 0.152 g
Glycine 0.038 g
Histidine 0.077 g
Isoleucine 0.028 g 2 %
Cystine 0.009 g
Lysine 0.050 g 2 %
Leucine 0.068 g 2 %
Phenylalanine 0.049 g 3 %
Methionine 0.008 g 1 %
Serine 0.040 g
Threonine 0.028 g 3 %
Proline 0.028 g
Tyrosine 0.009 g 1 %
Tryptophan 0.009 g 3 %
Valine 0.047 g 3 %

## Carbohydrates

Carbohydrate 22.84 g 8 %
Sugars 12.23 g
Fiber 2.6 g 10 %

Glucose (dextrose) 4.98 g

Fructose 4.85 g

Starch 5.38 g

Maltose 0.01 g

Sucrose 2.39 g

**Fats and Fatty Acids**

Fat 0.33 g 1 %

Decanoic acid 0.001 g

Dodecanoic acid 0.002 g

Hexadecanoic acid 0.102 g

Octadecanoic acid 0.005 g

Saturated fatty acids 0.112 g 1 %

Monounsaturated fatty acids 0.032 g

Tetradecanoic acid 0.002 g

Octadecenoic acid 0.022 g

Hexadecenoic acid 0.010 g

Polyunsaturated fatty acids 0.073 g

Octadecadienoic acid 0.046 g

Octadecatrienoic acid 0.027 g

**Sterols**

Phytosterols 16.00 mg

**Others**

Water 74.91 g

Ash 0.82 g

# Chapter Three

## Health benefits of banana

*The following are several health benefits of banana.*

### A.  It prevents stroke and heart attack

Potassium helps for proper functioning of the heart and blood pressure regulation. A great amount of potassium can be found in banana. A healthy diet with banana combined a good lifestyle lowers the risk of heart attack and stroke.

Potassium content in bananas also helps the kidneys and bones in the body. Increase in potassium intake reduces calcium excretion in the urine which prevents painful kidney stones from occurring.

Banana intake once or twice in a day lowers the risk of brittle bones and osteoporosis.

### B.  It increases energy

A great source of energy is banana. It contains natural sugars and soluble fiber which provides a stable energy.

Banana boosts the vitamins and minerals in the body and also gives great energy.

## C.  It enhances digestion and treats constipation

Fiber is a necessary requirement for food to move easily through the digestive tract. It also enhances bowel movements. The high fiber in bananas helps to normalize bowel motility.

Dietary fiber can be found in banana. Bananas stimulate the development of good bacteria in the bowel.

Also, they produce digestive enzymes to enable the absorption of these nutrients. Occasional constipation can also be treated by regular consumption of bananas.

## D.  It can cure ulcers & heartburn

Banana contains fiber which enables food to move faster through your digestive tract preventing reflux. Bananas provide relief from acid reflux, heartburn and GERD.

They relieve stomach ulcers by coating the stomach lining against corrosive acids. Regular intake of bananas prevents stomach ulcers. The protective mucus barrier of the stomach becomes thick; preventing damage from hydrochloric acid.

Banana also contains protease inhibitors which eliminates stomach bacteria that causes ulcer.

## E.  It maintains proper level of blood sugar

Vitamin B6 can be found in banana. This vitamin is very important for the creation of hemoglobin for a healthy blood. Vitamin B6 helps to maintain a proper blood sugar level.

## F.  It gives a good skin condition

Banana peelings have great health benefits. They can be used for treating acne and psoriasis.

The inside of a freshly peeled banana skin should be rubbed over the affected area of the skin till the residue gets absorbed. The banana skin has a fatty acid content which relieves different skin conditions. It also acts as a great moisturizer.

The banana peels treatment also heals warts. A Rub a small piece of banana peel over the affected area, hold it tightly in place. It is advisable to leave it on the affected spot overnight and repeated severally for a week or till the period the wart disappears.

## G.  It can prevent cancer

A research carried out in Japan revealed that bananas which are fully ripe and contain dark spots can be traced to the production of TNF–a compound. This compound has the ability to increase white blood cell production, thus improving immunity and fighting cancerous cell changes.

## H.  It improves your mood and reduces stress

Banana contains amino acid tryptophan. This nutrient is usually converted to serotonin by the body. A happy mood-brain neurotransmitter is serotonin.

Proper serotonin levels enhances your mood, improves your look and happiness levels. Serotonin also regulates sleep patterns.

Bananas supply tryptophan to your system. When stressed, try to eat two or more bananas.

## I.  It cures hangover

For those who have drunk so much the past night, blend some banana with berries, cow's milk or coconut milk and ice. The mixture is a very good hangover recovery drink.

## J.  It  fights against muscle cramps

Bananas when eaten prevent muscle cramps during sport activities or work outs. It also protects against night time leg cramps.

## K.  It can counteract the loss of calcium and also build strong bones

During urination, bananas tend to counteract calcium loss. And also, strong bones are being built when bananas are consumed regularly.

## L.   Bananas protect against type 11 diabetes

Regular consumption of bananas help the body resists type 11 diabetes.

## M.   It strengthens the blood and relieves anemia

The iron in banana strengthens the blood and relieves anemia.

## N. It protects against stroke and heart attack

Bananas contain a high quantity of potassium and a low quantity of salt, therefore it lowers blood pressure and also protect against stroke and heart attack.

## O. It prevents cancer of the kidney and eye macular degeneration

A regular intake of banana prevents kidney cancer and macular degeneration of the eyes.

## P. It contains calcium which builds strong bones

Bananas contain calcium which builds strong bones in the body when consumed frequently.

## Q. It makes you mentally sharp

Frequent consumption of banana makes you mentally sharper because it contains potassium.

**R. It protects against chronic diseases**

Bananas are high in antioxidants. These antioxidants protect from free radicals and chronic diseases.

**S. It reduces nausea and gives balance to blood sugar level**

In between meals consume two or more bananas; this stabilizes blood sugar and reduces nausea often caused by morning sickness.

**T. It relieves itching and irritation**

The inside of a banana peel can be used to relieve itching and irritation of a bug bite or hives. Just rub the peel gently on the affected area.

**U. It controls blood sugar**

A healthy diet containing banana helps to control blood sugar level.

## V. It lowers body temperature

Eating banana lowers body temperature on a hot day or when ill with fever.

## W. It deals with smoking withdrawal symptoms

Bananas contain high levels of magnesium, B-vitamins and potassium which deal effectively with smoking withdrawal symptoms.

## X. It can be used as a polish

Rub the inside of a banana peel on leather shoes and polish using a dry cloth.

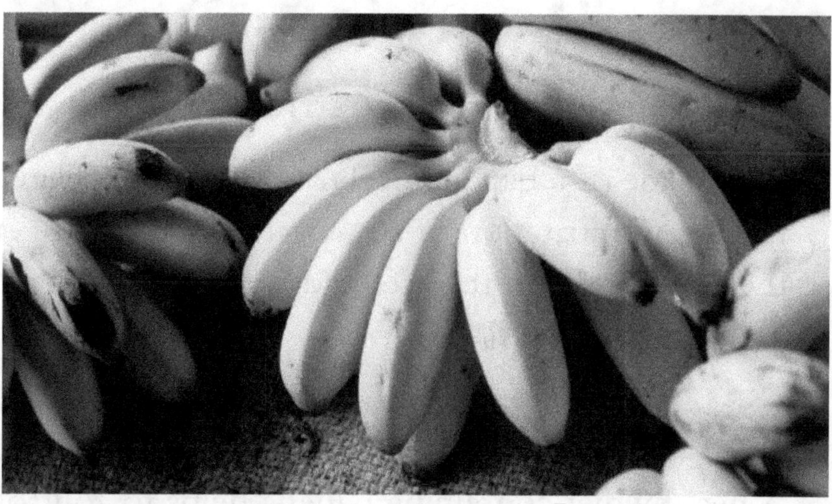

# Chapter four

## Banana Smoothie

Banana can be mixed with other ingredients to produce a very nutritious smoothie good for the body.

A banana smoothie can be prepared this way:

> 2 bananas (fresh or frozen)
> 1 1/2 cups of almond milk
> 1/2 tsp of ground cinnamon
> 1/2 avocado
> 1 tsp of raw honey
> 1 tsp of chia seeds
> 1 tsp of bee pollen
> 1/2 tsp of vanilla paste
> 1 tsp of Super food Protein (optional)
> 1 tsp of peanut butter (optional)
> Handful of ice

## Method of preparation

All ingredients should be placed in a blender. Blend for about sixty seconds till it becomes smooth.

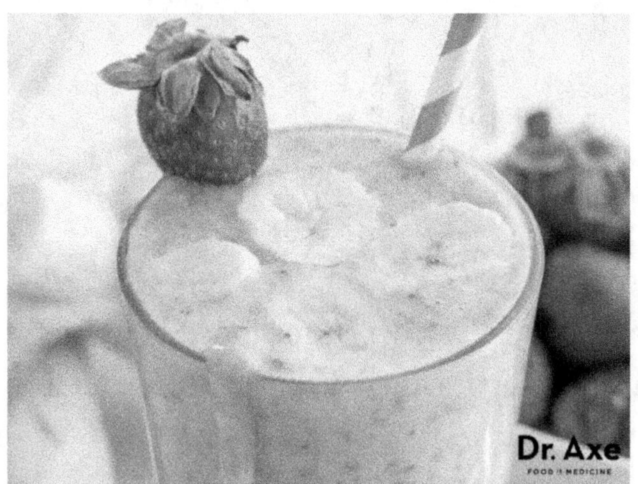
Dr. Axe
FOOD IS MEDICINE

# Chapter five

## Summary/Key points

1. It is edible.
2. It contains several nutrients.
3. It prevents stroke and heart attack.
4. It cures ulcer and heartburn.
5. Proper regulation of blood sugar level.
6. It fights against cancer.
7. It fights against type 11 diabetes.
8. It builds strong bones.
9. It prevents kidney cancer and eye macular degeneration.
10. It strengthens the blood.
11. It causes mental sharpness.
12. It deals effectively with smoking withdrawal symptoms.
13. It can be used for a smoothie.

The health benefits of banana fruit cannot be over emphasized. It is highly nutritious and extremely good for the health of the body. It effectively prevents most chronic diseases that fight against the body.

Frequent intake of banana will bring great health to the body. It is a must added fruit to each and every diet.

# Conclusion

As explained earlier in this book; banana is a great fruit with several health benefits. It can help combat depression, treat constipation and diarrhea, ulcers and heartburn, make you mentally sharp, relieve nausea caused by morning sickness, cure hangovers, protect against cancer of the kidney, diabetes, osteoporosis, blindness, etc.

Next time you see a bright colorful green or yellow fruit, it is none other than banana, one of the healthiest fruits on planet earth.

ABOUT THE AUTHOR

Mercy Obidake is a Writer, TV presenter, and blogger. She writes scripts for movies and Television programs, novels, articles and eBooks.

Aside from writing, she enjoys providing humanitarian services to the less privileged in society.